5:2 Diet

Intermittent Fasting Recipes for Beginners

PLUS 5 WEEKS MEAL PLAN FOR WEIGHT CONTROL

Stefany H. Lawrence

Table of Contents

Introduction

I want to thank you and congratulate you for downloading the book, "*5:2 Diet: Intermittent Fasting Recipes for Beginners – PLUS 5 WEEKS MEAL PLAN FOR WEIGHT CONTROL.*"

This book contains proven steps and strategies on how to follow the 5:2 Diet.

In this book, you will discover the simple three-step strategy on how you can follow the 5:2 Diet. Learn about how the days for "fast" and "feast" work, and how easy it is to follow the 5:2 Diet for weight loss and management.

Acquire a 5-week meal plan filled with delicious, easy-to-prepare and, most importantly, nutritious recipes for intermittent fasting. You will find over 40 delicious breakfast, main dish, side dish, and snack recipes, all of which are incorporated into the 5-week meal plan.

This book is for anyone who wants to lose weight in a healthy, sustainable, and enjoyable way. Learn more about the 5:2 Diet by turning to Chapter 1 right now!

Thanks again for downloading this book, I hope you enjoy it!

Chapter 1 – The 5:2 Diet Basics

The 5:2 Diet is pretty straightforward: eat regularly for five days and "fast" for two days. This is the basic rule that you follow every week. But of course, there are more details to the diet than just that. Here is the breakdown:

Two Days of "Fasting"

The reason why the word "fast" is enclosed in quotation marks is that you are not really going to be starving yourself for 48 hours. Rather, you are to eat only a quarter of the amount that your body normally needs. These should be in the form of light meals and should be consumed no more than three times per day.

The best part about the fasting days is that you do not have to go through them for two consecutive days. You can instead schedule them days apart. For example, if you want to fast on Saturday, you can schedule the second fast on Wednesday. This strategy is actually recommended to beginners so that they can avoid suffering from cravings that often lead to binge eating.

However, if you really prefer to *fast* – as in, consume nothing but water, tea, juices, or smoothies – then you are free to do so. That is, unless your doctor told you not to. Those who should *never* consider the 5:2 diet at all are children and teenagers (you still need those nutrients to grow up healthy and strong), pregnant and lactating women, and those who have a history of eating disorders. Those who have an existing medical condition such as diabetes should consult their doctor before trying this diet.

Five Days of "Feasting"

Technically, you are not really going to go "all out" for five days, especially if your goal is to lose weight. The word "feast" in the 5:2 Diet is mainly for hype purposes. Rather, it means you can eat whatever you want just as long as the amount suits your daily needs. Naturally, you would want to nourish your body with different nutrients during the "feast" days so you should choose nutritious, low calorie food.

When it comes to the number of meals you should eat during the "feast" days, the answer would depend on your lifestyle. The general rule is to eat three regular meals (breakfast, lunch, and dinner) with a snack in between.

However, it would be more important to just rely on the "eat until you are 80 percent satisfied" rule. Each person has different needs, and those who live a sedentary lifestyle should generally eat less than those who are quite active most of the time. Nevertheless, it helps to keep healthy snacks in store just in case you get hungry. That way, you will not end up running to the nearest fast food restaurant and gorging on high calorie, low nutrient meals.

In a nutshell, the 5:2 Diet is about eating healthy and controlling your portions. For five days, eat as you normally would. For two days, eat a lot less or not at all. Choose healthy food as often as possible and build the right habits to make this diet sustainable, natural, and enjoyable for you.

Chapter 2 – The Three-Step Plan to Start the 5:2 Diet

So, are you ready to start the 5:2 Diet? If this is your first time, then not to worry for you will find three concrete steps to implementing this diet every day. After reading the steps, you can then head on over to Chapter 3 for the 5-week meal plan.

Ready? Let's start:

Step 1: Start a Diet and Fitness Journal.

Your journal will be where you will keep a record of all the important information regarding your weight loss and overall health journey.

On the first page, write the date and then the following details: your age, sex, height, and weight. You can even include additional facts such as your blood sugar and cholesterol levels, and whatever else you wish to measure.

It is also important to write down in your journal any food allergies you may have, or foods you wish to cut out of your diet such as soft drinks, alcohol, and deep-fried food. Then, write down the foods you would like to eat more of, such as leafy greens and organic seafood or meat.

Finally, your journal is where you should write down your goals. Make sure that you specify them in that you should not just say "I want to lose weight." Rather, say something like: "I want to consume half a plate full of vegetables first in each meal." Make sure to include a "start" date next to each goal. Add an "end" date if it's applicable as well.

Step 2: Determine How Many Calories You Need.

Your Basal Metabolic Rate – or BMR for short – is the number of calories your body needs to stay alive. It is determined based on your age, height, sex, current weight, and activity level. There are plenty of online calculators for BMR, so you should simply pull one up online and type in your details.

For example, the BMR of a 27-year-old woman who is 5 feet 1 inch tall, weighs 127.6 pounds, and does no exercise whatsoever is **1,127 calories.** This means she needs to eat less than that if she wants to lose weight, or more if she wants to gain weight.

Once you have identified your BMR, you can add more calories to it as well, especially if you are going to be doing a lot of physical activities on certain days. While you do not necessarily have to count calories every single time, it does help to have an idea of how much your body needs so that you can avoid overeating or not eating enough.

Step 3: Create your 5:2 Diet Meal Plan Based on Your Daily Caloric Needs

After you have determined your caloric needs, the final step is to choose your two "fast" days and five "feast" days within each week.

For instance, some people prefer to do the "feast" days on the weekdays because they need the added energy for work. Then, they would simply "fast" on the weekends as they will be staying at home.

Others prefer to separate their two "fast" days so that they would not feel overwhelmed by their hunger cravings. For example, the first fast day can be on a Thursday, while the second one is on a Sunday.

However you plan your fast and feast days, you must lay them out on a sheet of paper and then choose what to have for each meal of each day. This is going to be your meal plan, and it will serve as your guide to keep you from binge eating on unhealthy foods during feast days, or to become tempted to "feast" when it is supposed to be your "fast" day.

To help get you started, you have an entire 5-week meal plan laid out for you in the next chapter.

Chapter 3 – The 5:2 Diet 5-week Meal Plan

Now that you know all about the 5:2 Diet, you can now move on to creating a personalized meal plan. Give yourself 5 weeks to really get into the 5:2 Diet so that you can build the habit of preparing your own meals as well as eating healthy food.

Below is a suggested 5-week meal plan that makes use of all the recipes in this book. Each week is divided into two categories: 5 "feast" days and 2 "fast" days. The suggested meals for feast days are breakfast, lunch, dinner, and at least one snack, while the ones for fast days are only the first three.

The amount of calories per serving for each meal is also included, that way you can adjust the amount of servings that is suitable to your caloric needs. For example, if you take a look at Week 1, "Feast" Day 1, you will notice that the grand total amount of calories is only 733. Naturally, you might need a lot more than that. So, you can either double the amount of servings for two or more dishes, or you can include your favorite healthy sides (such as steamed vegetables, rice, whole wheat dinner rolls, and so on) to add more calories.

For fast days, you may choose to follow the meal plan or, if you are adamant about it and if your doctor has given you his or her approval, you may choose to eat much less.

You might notice that certain dishes are served again within the same week, and the reason is that this meal plan is meant for making meals ahead of time. In other words, you are encouraged to do grocery shopping and cook in bulk on the first day (ideally your rest day, such as Sunday). Then, the food can be stored in airtight containers and refrigerated so that all you will have to do is reheat and serve. This helps significantly reduce the amount of time you need to spend on cooking and cleaning up, therefore encouraging you to prepare your own healthy meals.

Overall, this meal plan is to help keep you from constantly worrying about what to have for each meal. It is also meant to help you become more conscious of your portions in terms of calories. Try to follow this meal plan for five consecutive weeks and you will definitely notice a positive difference in your body and overall health.

But before you begin, it is of absolute importance that you consult your doctor, especially if you have a medical condition, such as type 2 diabetes. There might be certain nutrients that you need more of but the meal plan does not cover. If so, you might either need to take supplements, or add or avoid certain ingredients. So, make sure to get your doctor's approval before you start.

Week 1

5-Day "Feast"

Day 1:

Breakfast: Banana Berry Oatmeal Milkshake (190 cal)

Lunch: Oriental Beef Stir Fry (200 cal)

Dinner: Roasted Lemon Fennel with Olives (230 cal)

Snack(s): Fruity Oat Bars (113 cal)

Day 2:

Breakfast: Mexican Egg Skillet (204 cal)

Lunch: Chicken and Veggie Stew (238 cal)

Dinner: Spiced Carrot and Parsnip Soup (200 cal)

Snack(s): Zesty Poached Pears (90 cal)

Day 3:

Breakfast: Brie and Bell Pepper Frittata (216 cal)

Lunch: Oriental Beef Stir Fry (200 cal)

Dinner: Roasted Lemon Fennel with Olives (230 cal)

Snack(s): Fruity Oat Bars (113 cal)

Day 4:

Breakfast: Banana Berry Oatmeal Milkshake (190 cal)

Lunch: Chicken and Veggie Stew (238 cal)

Dinner: Spiced Carrot and Parsnip Soup (200 cal)

Snack(s): Zesty Poached Pears (90 cal)

Day 5:

Breakfast: Mexican Egg Skillet (204 cal)

Lunch: Sweet and Sour Beef Salad (230 cal)

Dinner: Roasted Lemon Fennel with Olives (230 cal)

Snack(s): Fruity Oat Bars (113 cal)

2-Day "Fast"

Day 1:

Breakfast: Fruity Yogurt Bowls (112 cal)

Lunch: Thai Shrimp and Rice Noodle Salad (171 cal)

Dinner: Ginger, Tomato and Chickpea Bowl (175 cal)

Day 2:

Breakfast: Baby Flapjacks and Smoked Salmon (136 cal)

Lunch: Hot Bean and Garlic Soup (159 cal)

Dinner: Fattoush (180 cal)

Week 2

5-Day "Feast"

Day 1:

Breakfast: Brie and Bell Pepper Frittata (216 cal)

Lunch: Sweet and Sour Beef Salad (230 cal)

Dinner: Roasted Tomato, Eggplant and Mozzarella (240 cal)

Snack(s): Zesty Poached Pears (90 cal)

Day 2:

Breakfast: Baked Basil Egg and Cheese Bites (231 cal)

Lunch: Southeast Asian Chicken Noodle Soup (229 cal)

Dinner: Roasted Vegetable Salad (240 cal)

Snack(s): Soft Almond Cookies (130 cal)

Day 3:

Breakfast: Cinnamon Banana Oatmeal Pancakes (340 cal)

Lunch: Cannellini Bean and Leek Spaghetti with Walnuts (379 cal)

Dinner: Roasted Tomato, Eggplant and Mozzarella (240 cal)

Snack(s): Warm Avocado, Grapefruit and Endive Snacks (225 cal)

Day 4:

Breakfast: Chickpea Pancakes with Blueberry Maple Sauce (343 cal)

Lunch: Southeast Asian Chicken Noodle Soup (229 cal)

Dinner: Roasted Vegetable Salad (240 cal)

Snack(s): Soft Almond Cookies (130 cal)

Day 5:

Breakfast: Brie and Bell Pepper Frittata (216 cal)

Lunch: Cannellini Bean and Leek Spaghetti with Walnuts (379 cal)

Dinner: Roasted Tomato, Eggplant and Mozzarella (240 cal)

Snack(s): Spiced Roasted Chickpeas (150 cal)

2-Day "Fast"

Day 1:

Breakfast: Cinnamon and Seed Oatmeal (137 cal)

Lunch: Shrimp and Spinach in Golden Sauce (162 cal)

Dinner: Orange and Fennel Salad (185 cal)

Day 2:

Breakfast: Blueberry Whole Wheat Muffins (175 cal)

Lunch: Mushroom Miso Stew (120 cal)

Dinner: Roasted Garlicky Tomatoes (185 cal)

Week 3

5-Day "Feast"

Day 1:

Breakfast: Chickpea Pancakes with Blueberry Maple Sauce (343 cal)

Lunch: Roasted Vegetable Lasagna (387 cal)

Dinner: Artichoke and Mushroom Soup (250 cal)

Snack(s): Warm Avocado, Grapefruit and Endive Snacks (225 cal)

Day 2:

Breakfast: Tex Mex Tofu Scramble (355 cal)

Lunch: Vegetable Korma (397 cal)

Dinner: Moroccan Couscous and Veggie Bowl (260 cal)

Snack(s): Spiced Roasted Chickpeas (150 cal)

Day 3:

Breakfast: Raspberry and Almond Butter Quesadilla (379 cal)

Lunch: Roasted Vegetable Lasagna (387 cal)

Dinner: Artichoke and Mushroom Soup (250 cal)

Snack(s): Cayenne Trail Mix (184 cal)

Day 4:

Breakfast: Chickpea Pancakes with Blueberry Maple Sauce (343 cal)

Lunch: Vegetable Korma (397 cal)

Dinner: Moroccan Couscous and Veggie Bowl (260 cal)

Snack(s): Spiced Roasted Chickpeas (150 cal)

Day 5:

Breakfast: Tex Mex Tofu Scramble (355 cal)

Lunch: Roasted Vegetable Lasagna (387 cal)

Dinner: Artichoke and Mushroom Soup (250 cal)

Snack(s): Cayenne Trail Mix (184 cal)

2-Day "Fast"

Day 1:

Breakfast: Fruity Yogurt Bowls (112 cal)

Lunch: Shrimp and Spinach in Golden Sauce (162 cal)

Dinner: Ginger, Tomato and Chickpea Bowl (175 cal)

Day 2:

Breakfast: Baby Flapjacks and Smoked Salmon (136 cal)

Lunch: Thai Shrimp and Rice Noodle Salad (171 cal)

Dinner: Fattoush (180 cal)

Week 4

5-Day "Feast"

Day 1:

Breakfast: Blueberry Whole Wheat Muffins (175 cal)

Lunch: Cheddar Barley and Butternut Squash Casserole (414 cal)

Dinner: Split Pea and Carrot Curry (260 cal)

Snack(s): Nutty Cherry Bombs (276 cal)

Day 2:

Breakfast: Banana Berry Oatmeal Milkshake (190 cal)

Lunch: Oriental Beef Stir Fry (200 cal)

Dinner: Split Pea and Carrot Curry (260 cal)

Snack(s): Zesty Baked Apples (163 cal)

Day 3:

Breakfast: Mexican Egg Skillet (204 cal)

Lunch: Cheddar Barley and Butternut Squash Casserole (414 cal)

Dinner: Split Pea and Carrot Curry (260 cal)

Snack(s): Nutty Cherry Bombs (276 cal)

Day 4:

Breakfast: Blueberry Whole Wheat Muffins (175 cal)

Lunch: Chicken and Veggie Stew (238 cal)

Dinner: Split Pea and Carrot Curry (260 cal)

Snack(s): Zesty Baked Apples (163 cal)

Day 5:

Breakfast: Mexican Egg Skillet (204 cal)

Lunch: Cheddar Barley and Butternut Squash Casserole (414 cal)

Dinner: Split Pea and Carrot Curry (260 cal)

Snack(s): Peanut Butter Muffins (184 cal)

2-Day "Fast"

Day 1:

Breakfast: Cinnamon and Seed Oatmeal (137 cal)

Lunch: Hot Bean and Garlic Soup (159 cal)

Dinner: Roasted Garlicky Tomatoes (185 cal)

Day 2:

Breakfast: Blueberry Whole Wheat Muffins (175 cal)

Lunch: Mushroom Miso Stew (120 cal)

Dinner: Orange and Fennel Salad (185 cal)

Week 5

5-Day "Feast"

Day 1:

Breakfast: Baked Basil Egg and Cheese Bites (231 cal)

Lunch: Oriental Beef Stir Fry (200 cal)

Dinner: Spiced Carrot and Parsnip Soup (200 cal)

Snack(s): Zesty Baked Apples (163 cal)

Day 2:

Breakfast: Cinnamon Banana Oatmeal Pancakes (340 cal)

Lunch: Chicken and Veggie Stew (238 cal)

Dinner: Roasted Lemon Fennel with Olives (230 cal)

Snack(s): Banana and Dark Chocolate Sandwiches (318 cal)

Day 3:

Breakfast: Chickpea Pancakes with Blueberry Maple Sauce (343 cal)

Lunch: Oriental Beef Stir Fry (200 cal)

Dinner: Spiced Carrot and Parsnip Soup (200 cal)

Snack(s): Cilantro and Hummus Quesadillas (193 cal)

Day 4:

Breakfast: Tex Mex Tofu Scramble (355 cal)

Lunch: Chicken and Veggie Stew (238 cal)

Dinner: Roasted Lemon Fennel with Olives (230 cal)

Snack(s): Almond Raspberry Yogurt Bowls (207 cal)

Day 5:

Breakfast: Raspberry and Almond Butter Quesadilla (379 cal)

Lunch: Sweet and Sour Beef Salad (230 cal)

Dinner: Roasted Tomato, Eggplant and Mozzarella (240 cal)

Snack(s): Cilantro and Hummus Quesadillas (193 cal)

2-Day "Fast"

Day 1:

Breakfast: Fruity Yogurt Bowls (112 cal)

Lunch: Shrimp and Spinach in Golden Sauce (162 cal)

Dinner: Fattoush (180 cal)

Day 2:

Breakfast: Baby Flapjacks and Smoked Salmon (136 cal)

Lunch: Thai Shrimp and Rice Noodle Salad (171 cal)

Dinner: Ginger, Tomato and Chickpea Bowl (175 cal)

Chapter 4 – Breakfast Recipes

Fruity Yogurt Bowls

Number of regular servings: 3

Calories per regular serving: 112

You will need:

- 2 cups cubed melon
- 1 cup sliced strawberries
- 1 ½ cups fresh berries, such as raspberries or blueberries
- ½ cup freshly squeezed orange or lemon juice
- 3 Tbsp non-fat Greek yogurt
- 3 tsp raw honey

How to Prepare:

Combine the melon, strawberries, and berries in a bowl. Add the orange or lemon juice and toss gently to coat. Set aside at room temperature for 30 minutes.

After 30 minutes, divide the yogurt among three bowls. Divide the fruit mixture between the servings, then drizzle the honey on top. Serve right away.

Chickpea Pancakes with Blueberry Maple Sauce

Number of regular servings: 6

Calories per regular serving: 343

You will need:

- 5 large eggs
- 2 bananas, sliced thinly
- 16 oz frozen blueberries
- 1 ½ cups plain Greek yogurt
- 1 ½ cups cooked chickpeas
- ¾ cup whole milk
- 1/3 cup all-purpose flour

- 1/3 cup pure maple syrup

- 1/3 tsp sea salt

- Nonstick cooking spray

How to Prepare:

Set the oven to 350 degrees F to preheat.

In a food processor, blend the eggs with 2 ½ tablespoons yogurt with 1 ½ tablespoons maple syrup, and milk. Add the salt and blend well until combined.

Pour in the flour and chickpeas, then blend until smooth. Set aside for 15 minutes.

Place a pancake griddle over medium high flame and heat through. Lightly sprits with nonstick cooking spray, then add a quarter cup of the batter on top.

Cook the pancake for 2 minutes per side, or until browned. Transfer to a platter and repeat with the remaining batter.

Blend 1 ½ cups of the blueberries until pasty, then add the remaining maple syrup and blend until smooth.

Spoon the blueberry mixture on top of the pancakes, then top with a dollop of yogurt and banana slices. Serve right away.

Baby Flapjacks and Smoked Salmon

Number of regular servings: 3

Calories per regular serving: 136

You will need:

- 2 small eggs
- ¾ cup all-purpose flour
- 3 Tbsp low fat milk
- 2 Tbsp water
- Sea salt and white pepper, to taste
- Cooking spray, as needed

For the Smoked Salmon

- 35 grams smoked salmon
- 3 Tbsp quark cheese
- 3 tsp chopped fresh chives
- 1 tsp freshly squeezed lemon juice

- Sea salt and freshly ground black pepper, to taste

How to Prepare:

Sift the flour into a mixing bowl, then add a dash of salt and white pepper. Mix well, then add the milk, eggs, and water. Mix well until just combined with a few lumps.

Lightly coat a pancake griddle with cooking spray, then place over medium flame. Add three tablespoons of the batter, then cook until firm and golden, about 2 minutes per side. Transfer to a plate and cook the remaining batter.

After cooking the flapjacks, combine the lemon juice and quark cheese in a bowl. Spoon the mixture over the flapjacks and add the smoked salmon on top. Garnish with chives and serve right away.

Brie and Bell Pepper Frittata

Number of regular servings: 6

Calories per regular serving: 216

You will need:

- 8 large eggs
- 1 shallot, minced
- 1 small garlic clove, minced
- 4 oz brie, chopped into chunks
- 1/3 cup chopped roasted red bell peppers
- 1/3 cup low fat milk
- 1/3 cup low fat plain Greek yogurt
- 1 ½ Tbsp olive oil
- ¾ tsp dried basil
- Garlic powder, to taste
- Sea salt and freshly ground black pepper, to taste

How to Prepare:

Set the oven to 400 degrees F to preheat.

Place a cast iron skillet over medium low flame and heat through. Once hot, add the olive oil and swirl to coat.

Stir in the shallot and sauté until translucent. Add the garlic and sauté for 30 seconds, or until fragrant.

Meanwhile, beat the eggs, milk, and yogurt in a bowl. Add the dried basil and then season with a pinch of garlic powder, salt, and pepper. Stir into the skillet and mix well with the shallot and garlic mixture.

Cover the skillet and cook over medium low flame for 5 minutes, or until the eggs are slightly firm. Transfer to the oven.

Bake for 12 minutes, or until golden brown and puffy. Transfer to a cooling rack and allow to cool slightly. Slice into wedges, then serve right away.

Blueberry Whole Wheat Muffins

Number of regular servings: 24 (muffins)

Calories per regular serving: 175

You will need:

- 2 eggs
- 2 cups low fat milk
- 1 ¼ cups whole wheat flour
- 1 ¼ cups all-purpose flour
- 1 cup fresh blueberries (or any other berry in season)
- ½ cup canola oil
- ¼ cup sifted confectioner's sugar
- ¼ cup soft brown sugar
- 2 Tbsp baking powder
- 2 tsp ground mixed spice
- 1 tsp sea salt

How to Prepare:

Combine half the blueberries with the confectioner's sugar, then toss to coat and set aside.

Set the oven to 350 degrees F to preheat.

Line 24 muffin tins with paper liners, then set aside.

Sift the flours into a bowl, then sift in the baking powder, salt, brown sugar, and mixed spice. Mix well and set aside.

Beat together the eggs, milk and oil in a separate bowl, then set aside.

Create a pit in the center of the flour mixture and add the egg mixture. Mix well until just combined, then fold in the sugar and blueberry mixture. Do not over-mix or the muffins will come out tough.

Divide the batter among the prepared muffin tins, then divide the remaining blueberries between servings.

Bake for 20 minutes, or until the muffins are completely puffed and firm. Transfer to a cooling rack and allow to cool. Best served warm.

Can be refrigerated for up to 5 days or frozen for up to 3 months.

Mexican Egg Skillet

Number of regular servings: 3

Calories per regular serving: 204

You will need:

- 3 eggs
- 1 small red bell pepper, seeded and chopped
- 3 spring onions, chopped
- ½ red chili pepper, seeded and minced
- 300 grams canned chopped tomatoes
- 1 ½ Tbsp chopped fresh coriander or parsley
- 1 ½ tsp balsamic vinegar
- 1 ½ tsp olive oil
- 1 ½ pieces whole wheat pita bread, lightly toasted
- Sea salt and freshly ground black pepper, to taste

How to Prepare:

Place a large skillet over medium flame and heat through. Once hot, add the olive oil and swirl to coat. Sauté the bell pepper, chili pepper, and spring onion for about 3 minutes, or until tender.

Stir in the chopped tomatoes and add the balsamic vinegar. Season lightly with salt and pepper to taste, then sauté until combined. Simmer for about 3 minutes, or until slightly thickened.

Reduce to low flame and create three pits in the mixture. Crack one egg at a time into a bowl, then slip it into the pit. Cover and cook for 3 to 5 minutes, or until the eggs are set.

Once cooked, top with chopped fresh coriander and parsley, then serve with the pita bread.

———————————————————————

Raspberry and Almond Butter Quesadilla

Number of regular servings: 4

Calories per regular serving: 379

You will need:

- 3 cups raspberries, sliced thinly
- 2/3 cup nonfat Greek yogurt
- ½ cup almond butter
- 2 Tbsp mascarpone cheese
- 2 tsp dark brown sugar
- 2 tsp brown sugar
- 1 tsp pure vanilla extract
- ½ tsp ground cinnamon
- 4 whole wheat tortillas

How to Prepare:

Set the oven to 375 degrees F to preheat. Line a baking sheet with parchment paper and set aside.

Combine the raspberries in a bowl with half the vanilla extract and all the brown sugar. Spread on the prepared baking sheet and bake for 15 minutes.

Meanwhile, mix together the yogurt, dark brown sugar, cinnamon, almond butter, and mascarpone cheese in a food processor. Blend until combined.

Spread the yogurt and almond butter mixture on half of each tortilla, then add the roasted raspberry mixture on top of the other half. Sandwich the halves together, then set aside.

If desired, toast before serving. Best served warm.

_____

Banana Berry Oatmeal Milkshake

Number of regular servings: 2

Calories per regular serving: 190

You will need:

- 1 banana, peeled and sliced
- 4 Tbsp rolled oats
- 1 cup frozen berry, any kind
- ½ cup low fat milk
- ½ cup low fat Greek yogurt

How to Prepare:

Combine all the ingredients in a blender. Cover and blend until smooth.

Pour into glasses and serve right away.

———————————————————

Baked Basil Egg and Cheese Bites

Number of regular servings: 9

Calories per regular serving: 231

You will need:

- 12 eggs
- 2 shallots, diced
- 2 small Roma tomatoes, diced
- 2 ¼ cups cubed baguette or sourdough bread
- 2 cups shredded low fat mozzarella cheese
- ¾ cup low fat plain Greek yogurt
- ¾ cup chopped basil leaves
- ¾ tsp baking powder
- ¾ tsp fine sea salt
- ¾ tsp garlic powder
- ¾ tsp onion powder
- 1/3 tsp freshly ground black pepper
- Nonstick cooking spray, as needed

How to Prepare:

Set the oven to 350 degrees F to preheat. Lightly coat 24 mini muffin tins with nonstick cooking spray, then set aside.

Beat the eggs with the spices, baking powder, salt, pepper, and yogurt until smooth. Beat in the mozzarella cheese, shallot, and basil.

Divide the cubed bread among the muffin tins, then divide the diced tomato on top of each. Divide the egg mixture as well, then bake for 32 minutes, or until golden brown and firm.

Transfer to a cooling rack and allow to cool completely. Best served warm.

———————————————————

Cinnamon and Seed Oatmeal

Number of regular servings: 3

Calories per regular serving: 137

You will need:

- 60 grams rolled oats

- 24 raisins

- 1 ½ cups water

- 6 Tbsp low fat Greek yogurt

- 3 tsp seeds, such as sunflower, sesame, or pumpkin seeds

- Ground cinnamon, to taste

How to Prepare:

Combine the rolled oats, water, seeds, and raisins in a saucepan. Place over high flame and bring to a boil.

Once boiling, reduce to medium low flame, cover, and simmer for 5 minutes or until thickened to a desired consistency.

Divide the oatmeal among three bowls, then add a dollop of yogurt and a dash of cinnamon. Serve right away.

Cinnamon Banana Oatmeal Pancakes

Number of regular servings: 4

Calories per regular serving: 340

You will need:

- 2 large ripe bananas, mashed
- 2 large eggs
- 1 cup low fat plain Greek yogurt
- 1 cup whole wheat flour
- ½ cup rolled oats
- 1/3 cup low fat buttermilk
- 2 Tbsp dark brown sugar
- 1 ½ Tbsp pure vanilla extract
- 2 tsp baking powder
- 1 tsp ground cinnamon
- ½ tsp ground nutmeg
- ¼ tsp fine sea salt

How to Prepare:

Combine the yogurt, buttermilk, banana, vanilla extract, eggs, and sugar in a bowl. Fold in the oats, then set aside.

In a separate bowl, sift the flour, cinnamon, nutmeg, baking powder, and salt. Gradually fold the flour mixture into the yogurt mixture until combined. Do not over-mix or the pancakes will come out rubbery.

Place the pancake griddle over medium flame to heat.

Ladle a quarter cup of the batter onto the hot griddle and cook for 3 minutes per side, or until firm. Transfer to a plate and repeat with the remaining batter.

Best served warm.

Tex Mex Tofu Scramble

Number of regular servings: 2

Calories per regular serving: 355

You will need:

- 2 corn tortillas, chopped
- 2 garlic cloves, minced
- 1 green bell pepper, seeded and diced
- 1 tomato, diced
- 7 oz extra firm tofu, crumbled
- ½ cup diced red onion
- 4 Tbsp crumbled feta cheese
- 1 Tbsp nutritional yeast
- 4 tsp olive oil
- ½ tsp chili powder
- ½ tsp cumin
- ¼ tsp turmeric
- ¼ tsp sea salt

How to Prepare:

Place a large skillet over medium flame and heat through. Add the olive oil and swirl to coat.

Stir in the onion and sauté until translucent, then stir in the garlic and sauté until fragrant.

Add the bell pepper, crumbled tofu, tomato, spices, and nutritional yeast. Sauté for 5 minutes or until the bell pepper is crisp tender.

Turn off the heat and fold in the feta and chopped tortilla. Mix well, then transfer to a serving plate. Best served right away.

———————————————————————

Chapter 5 – Main Dish Recipes

Cheddar Barley and Butternut Squash Casserole

Number of regular servings: 9

Calories per regular serving: 414

You will need:

- 3 garlic cloves, minced
- 1 small red onion, minced
- 5 cups cubed butternut squash
- 4 ½ cups water
- 3 cups low fat milk
- 1 ½ cups shredded extra sharp cheddar cheese
- 1 ½ cups uncooked pearl barley
- 1 cup shredded Parmesan cheese
- 3 Tbsp olive oil

- 3 Tbsp grass fed butter

- 3 Tbsp all-purpose flour

- 3 tsp dried rosemary

- ¾ tsp fine sea salt

- 1/3 tsp freshly ground black pepper

- 1/6 tsp nutmeg

How to Prepare:

Set the oven to 350 degrees F to preheat.

Pour the water into a pot and stir in the barley. Place over high flame and bring to a boil. Once boiling, reduce to a simmer and cook, covered, for 40 minutes or until the barley has absorbed most of the water. Drain excess water, if needed.

Meanwhile, place a large skillet over medium high flame and heat through. Once hot, add the olive oil and swirl to coat. Sauté the onion until translucent, then stir in the garlic and sauté until fragrant.

Stir in the butternut squash and sauté for 10 minutes, or until fork tender.

Place a saucepan over medium flame and heat through. Once hot, add the butter, then stir in the flour and mix well until pasty. Add the milk, rosemary, nutmeg, salt, and pepper, then bring to a boil, stirring well. Continue stirring for about 5 minutes, or until thickened.

Turn off the heat and add the cheddar. Stir well until thoroughly combined.

In a large casserole, pour in the barley, then add the butternut squash mixture and Cheddar mixture. Stir well until combined, then add the Parmesan on top. Cover the casserole with a lid or aluminum foil, then bake for 25 minutes.

Uncover and set the oven to broil. Bake for an additional 5 minutes, or until golden brown.

Transfer to a cooling rack and let stand for 10 minutes. Best served warm.

Hot Bean and Garlic Soup

Number of regular servings: 3

Calories per regular serving: 159

You will need:

- 115 grams dried cannellini beans
- 2 garlic cloves, peeled
- 1 ½ Tbsp olive oil
- 1 Tbsp chopped fresh parsley
- Sea salt and black pepper, to taste

How to Prepare:

Place the dried beans in a bowl and add enough cold water to cover them by about an inch. Cover and soak for 8 hours (overnight).

The following day, drain the beans and place in a pot. Add enough water to cover them by about a quarter of an inch, then place over high flame and cover. Bring to a boil, then reduce to a simmer. Simmer for 25 to 30 minutes, or until tender.

Meanwhile, slice one garlic into thin slivers and mince the other.

Ladle half the beans into a blender or food processor and blend until smooth. Stir back into the pot.

Place a skillet over medium flame and heat half the olive oil. Cook the chopped garlic until golden brown, then pour into the bean soup and stir. Season to taste with salt and pepper.

Heat the remaining oil in the skillet and add the garlic slivers. Cook until golden brown, then turn off the heat.

Divide the soup into three servings, then top with the garlic slivers and parsley. Serve right away.

Chicken and Veggie Stew

Number of regular servings: 4

Calories per regular serving: 238

You will need:

- 4 skinless, boneless chicken breasts
- 4 small carrots, peeled and diced
- 1 small onion, chopped
- 4 cups chicken broth
- 1 cup chopped broccoli florets
- ½ Tbsp olive oil
- ¼ Tbsp freshly grated lemon zest
- 2 rosemary sprigs
- Sea salt and freshly ground black pepper, to taste

How to Prepare:

Wash the chicken breasts thoroughly, then blot dry with paper towels.

Score the chicken breasts all over with a sharp knife, then rub a teaspoon of olive oil all over. Rub the rosemary and lemon zest all over, then set aside.

Place a saucepan over medium flame and heat through. Once hot, add the remaining oil and swirl to coat. Cook the chicken for 5 minutes per side, or until cooked through and golden brown.

Pour the broth into the saucepan, then bring to a boil. Once boiling, reduce to low flame, cover, and simmer for 12 minutes.

Add the onion, carrot, and broccoli, then cover and cook for 3 minutes, or until the carrots and broccoli are tender.

Season to taste with salt and pepper, then divide into four servings and serve right away.

Shrimp and Spinach in Golden Sauce

Number of regular servings: 3

Calories per regular serving: 162

You will need:

- 1 small onion, sliced
- ½ inch fresh ginger, peeled and chopped
- 550 grams large shrimp
- 3 cups spinach
- 1 cup low fat coconut milk
- 1 ½ Tbsp vegetable oil
- 1 Tbsp freshly squeezed lime or lemon juice
- ¾ Tbsp black mustard seeds
- 1 ½ tsp ground turmeric
- ¾ tsp chili powder
- Ground cloves, to taste
- Sea salt, to taste

How to Prepare:

Pull off the heads of the shrimp, then de-vein. Leave the tail ends attached. Wash and drain, then blot dry with paper towels and set aside.

Place a saucepan over medium flame. Heat through, then add the oil and swirl to coat. Sauté the onion, ginger, and garlic until tender, then add the spices with a pinch of salt and ground cloves. Sauté until fragrant.

Pour in the coconut milk, then bring to a boil. Once boiling, reduce to a simmer. Let simmer for 3 minutes, then add the shrimp. Cook for 4 minutes or until the shrimp is almost cooked through.

Add the spinach, then stir and reduce to low flame. Cover and cook until the spinach is wilted.

Turn off the heat, then pour in the lime and lemon juice. Stir and serve right away.

Vegetable Korma

Number of regular servings: 6

Calories per regular serving: 397

You will need:

- 6 medium tomatoes, chopped
- 2 small white onions, chopped
- 1 ½ cups chopped cauliflower florets
- 1 ½ cups chopped carrot
- 1 ½ cups chopped zucchini
- 1 ½ cups chopped green beans or lima beans
- 1 ½ cups basmati rice
- ¾ cup coconut milk
- 6 Tbsp golden raisins
- 4 ½ Tbsp minced fresh ginger
- 3 Tbsp toasted slivered almonds
- 3 Tbsp canola oil
- 1 ½ tsp curry powder

- 1 ¼ tsp ground cardamom

- Sea salt and freshly ground black pepper, to taste

How to Prepare:

Prepare the rice based on package instructions. Set aside.

Combine the onion, ginger, and tomatoes in a food processor, then blend until pasty.

Place a saucepan over medium flame and heat through. Once hot, add the canola oil and swirl to coat. Stir in the curry powder and ground cardamom and sauté for about 30 seconds, or until fragrant.

Stir in the tomato puree and raisins, then let simmer until thickened.

Stir in the vegetables and coconut milk, then season to taste with salt and pepper.

Cover and simmer over medium low flame for about 6 minutes, or until the vegetables are fork tender.

Divide the rice into six servings, then divide the vegetable korma on top. Garnish with slivered almonds, then serve right away.

Oriental Beef Stir Fry

Number of regular servings: 3

Calories per regular serving: 200

You will need:

- ½ lb fillet steak, sliced into extra thin strips
- 2 spring onions, chopped
- 1 orange bell pepper, seeded and chopped into thin strips
- ½ red chili pepper, seeded and diced
- 2 cups chopped broccoli florets
- 1 ½ cups chopped bok choy or spinach
- ¾ Tbsp chili oil

For the Beef Marinade:

- 1 inch fresh ginger, peeled and diced
- 1 ½ Tbsp black bean paste
- 1 ½ Tbsp yellow bean paste
- 1 ½ Tbsp sherry vinegar

- ¾ Tbsp dark soy sauce

How to Prepare:

Combine all the ingredients for the marinade in a bowl, then add the beef strips. Toss well to coat. Cover and refrigerate for 1 to 8 hours.

After marinating, transfer the beef to a bowl; reserve the marinade. Place a wok over high flame and heat through. Once hot, add the oil and swirl to coat. And swirl to coat.

Stir fry the beef for 4 minutes, then add the vegetables and stir fry everything for 4 minutes.

Pour in the marinade and simmer until thickened. Transfer to a plate and serve right away.

Cannellini Bean and Leek Spaghetti with Walnuts

Number of regular servings: 4

Calories per regular serving: 379

You will need:

- 1 garlic cloves, minced
- 12 oz canned cannellini beans, rinsed and drained thoroughly
- 8 oz whole wheat or gluten-free spaghetti
- 2 oz crumbled feta cheese
- 4 cups chopped leeks
- ¾ cup vegetable broth
- ¾ cup chopped yellow bell pepper
- ¼ cup chopped toasted walnuts
- ¾ Tbsp olive oil
- Red pepper flakes, to taste
- Sea salt and freshly ground black pepper, to taste

How to Prepare:

Boil the spaghetti based on manufacturer's instructions. Drain well and set aside.

Place a saucepan over medium high flame and heat through. Add the oil and swirl to coat. Sauté the bell pepper and leek with a pinch of red pepper flakes for about 8 minutes.

Once the leeks and bell pepper are tender, stir in the garlic, beans, and broth. Set to low flame and simmer for 5 minutes.

Divide the cooked spaghetti into four portions, then ladle the sauce on top. Garnish with walnuts and feta cheese, then serve right away.

Sweet and Sour Beef Salad

Number of regular servings: 3

Calories per regular serving: 230

You will need:

- 200 grams fillet steak
- 3 cups salad greens
- ¾ Tbsp crushed black peppercorns
- ¾ Tbsp sesame seeds
- ¾ tsp ground coriander
- ¾ tsp freshly ground black pepper
- 1/6 tsp Chinese five spice
- 1 lime

For the Dressing:

- 2 shallots, peeled
- 3 garlic cloves, peeled
- 1 large chili, seeded
- 1 inch fresh ginger, peeled

- 1 lemon grass stalk, chopped
- 1 lime, sliced into wedges
- 2 Tbsp sunflower oil
- ¾ Tbsp tamarind paste
- ¾ Tbsp light soy sauce
- 1 ½ tsp brown sugar
- ¾ tsp cumin seeds
- Sea salt, to taste

How to Prepare:

Set the oven to 400 degrees F to preheat.

Wash the steak thoroughly, then blot dry with paper towels and set aside.

Combine the crushed black peppercorns with the black pepper, five spice, and ground coriander. Rub the mixture all over the steak, then cover and refrigerate for 2 hours.

In the meantime, prepare the dressing. Combine the lemongrass, garlic, ginger, chilies, and shallot in a roasting pan. Add the cumin seeds, then drizzle the oil on top. Toss well to combine.

Roast the mixture in the oven for about 25 minutes, or until tender and browned. Set aside on a cooling rack and allow to cool.

Once cooled, transfer the roasted herb mixture into the food processor and add the soy sauce, tamarind paste, and brown sugar. Blend until pasty, adding more water if needed. Season to taste with salt.

Lightly coat a skillet with oil, then place over medium high flame. Once hot, sear the steak for about 1 minute per side, pressing down hard on the steak with a spatula.

Transfer the beef to a plate and let rest for 2 minutes. Slice thinly.

Divide the greens among three plates, then add the thinly sliced beef on top of the greens. Drizzle the dressing on top, then garnish with sesame seeds and lime wedges. Serve right away.

_____

Roasted Vegetable Lasagna

Number of regular servings: 9

Calories per regular serving: 387

You will need:

- 1 large zucchini, sliced thinly
- 1 yellow onion, sliced thinly
- 2 bell peppers, seeded and sliced thinly
- 12 oz thinly sliced white mushrooms
- 1 ½ Tbsp olive oil
- 1/3 tsp fine sea salt
- 1/3 tsp freshly ground black pepper
- 12 whole wheat or gluten-free lasagna noodles

For the Filling:

- 3 garlic cloves, minced
- 21 oz extra firm tofu
- ¾ cup roasted cashews
- 1/3 cup nutritional yeast

- 1 ½ tsp dried basil

- 1 ½ tsp dried oregano

- 1/3 tsp fine sea salt

For the Sauce:

- 3 garlic cloves, minced

- 32 oz canned crushed tomatoes

- 3 Tbsp tomato paste

- 1 ½ Tbsp olive oil

- 1 ½ tsp dried oregano

- 1 ½ tsp dried basil

- ¾ tsp fine sea salt

- 1/3 tsp crushed red pepper flakes

How to Prepare:

Cook the lasagna noodles based on manufacturer's instructions. Drain and set aside.

Make the filling. Place the cashews in a bowl, then add boiling water until covered. Set aside for 45 minutes to soak.

Once the cashews are soaked, drain and place in a food processor. Add the garlic, basil, oregano, salt, and nutritional yeast. Blend until combined, then pour into a bowl and set aside.

Add the tofu and crumble well with the cashew mixture. Mix well and set aside.

Roast the vegetables by placing them in a baking sheet and adding the olive oil. Season with the salt and pepper, then toss well to coat.

Spread out into a single layer, then roast for 15 to 20 minutes, or until tender. Set on a cooling rack. Reduce the oven temperature to 350 degrees F.

Make the sauce by placing a saucepan over medium flame. Once hot, add the olive oil and swirl to coat. Stir in the garlic and sauté until fragrant. Add the tomato paste, tomatoes, oregano, basil, salt, and pepper.

Bring to a boil, then reduce to low flame and cover. Simmer for 12 minutes.

To prepare the lasagna, spread 1/3 cup of sauce into a large baking dish, then add a layer of lasagna noodles.

Add a third of the tofu mixture on top, followed by a third of the roasted vegetables. Add some more sauce, then place some more noodles. Keep repeating until all the ingredients are used up, with the final layer being the sauce.

Cover the baking dish with aluminum foil, then bake for 40 minutes.

Uncover and bake for an additional 10 minutes, then transfer to a cooling rack and let set for about 12 minutes before slicing. Best served warm.

Southeast Asian Chicken Noodle Soup

Number of regular servings: 4

Calories per regular serving: 229

You will need:

- 2 skinless, chicken thighs, bone in
- 2 lemon grass stalks, rinsed and sliced thinly
- 2 inches fresh ginger, peeled and sliced
- 2 garlic cloves, sliced
- 1 to 2 red chilies, sliced
- 100 grams egg noodles
- 2 carrots, peeled and sliced into sticks
- ½ red bell pepper, seeded and chopped into strips
- 7 ½ cups water
- 2 cups chopped broccoli
- 1 ½ cups bean sprouts
- 2 Tbsp miso paste
- 2 tsp sesame oil

- 2 spring onions, chopped

How to Prepare:

Place the chicken, ginger, garlic, lemon grass, and chili in a pot and add 5 cups of water. Cover and place over high flame. Bring to a boil, then reduce to low flame and simmer for 20 minutes, or until the chicken is cooked through.

Transfer the chicken into a bowl, then set aside.

Pour the stock through a strainer and discard the solids. Return to the pot and add an additional 2 ½ cups of water.

Shred the chicken and stir the meat into the pot. Stir in the bell pepper, bean sprouts, and miso paste, then place over medium flame. Simmer until the vegetables are tender and the chicken is heated through.

Divide the soup into four servings, then top with sesame oil and spring onion. Serve right away.

———————————————————

Mushroom Miso Stew

Number of regular servings: 4

Calories per regular serving: 120

You will need:

- 3 dried shiitake mushrooms
- 1 green onion, chopped
- 1 small sweet potato, peeled and diced
- 1 inch fresh ginger, sliced into thin rounds
- 1 ½ pieces kombu seaweed
- 6 oz diced extra firm tofu
- 3 ½ cups water
- 1 ½ cups chopped green beans
- ¾ cup sliced button mushrooms
- ½ cup chopped leek
- 3 Tbsp miso paste
- 1 Tbsp low sodium soy sauce
- ¾ Tbsp rice wine vinegar

How to Prepare:

Pour the water into a saucepan, then add the shiitake mushrooms, ginger, rice wine vinegar, and soy sauce. Place over high flame and bring to a boil.

Once boiling, cover and reduce to medium low flame. Simmer for 10 minutes, then discard the ginger and shiitake mushrooms. Remove and chop the kombu, then set aside.

Stir the leek and button mushrooms into the soup, then cover and simmer over medium low flame. Simmer for 5 minutes, then add the green beans, kombu, and sweet potato.

Simmer for 5 minutes, or until the sweet potato is fork tender. Add the tofu and stir for 3 minutes. Turn off the heat and set aside.

Ladle about a cup of the broth into a bowl and stir in the miso paste. Stir the mixture into the soup and mix well. Top with green onion and serve right away.

Thai Shrimp and Rice Noodle Salad

Number of regular servings: 3

Calories per regular serving: 171

You will need:

- ¾ fresh shiitake mushrooms, trimmed and sliced
- 150 grams large shrimp, cooked, peeled and deveined
- 40 g dried rice noodles, chopped into bite-sized pieces
- 1 medium carrot, peeled and julienned
- 1 small zucchini, peeled and julienned
- 1 ½ Tbsp chopped fresh coriander
- ¾ Tbsp toasted sesame seeds

For the Dressing:

- 1 large garlic clove, crush
- 1 ½ Tbsp brown sugar
- ¾ Tbsp light soy sauce

- ¾ Tbsp wine vinegar

- ¾ Tbsp sesame oil

- ½ red chili, seeded and sliced

How to Prepare:

Prepare the dressing by placing the garlic in a bowl with the soy sauce, wine vinegar, sugar, and sesame oil. Stir in the chili slices, then set aside.

Cook the noodles based on package instructions, then drain and rinse under cold running water. Drain thoroughly, then transfer to a bowl and set aside.

Place the mushrooms into a bowl, then pour in the dressing and toss well to coat. Pour the mushroom and dressing mixture over the noodles, then lay the zucchini and carrot on top. Add the cooked shrimp, then toss everything to combine.

Top with coriander and sesame seeds, then serve right away.

Chapter 6 – Light Meal Recipes

Artichoke Heart, Tomato, Arugula and Chickpea Salad

Number of regular servings: 6

Calories per regular serving: 345

You will need:

- 9 oz jarred artichoke hearts in water, rinsed, drained and chopped
- 3 oz crumbled feta cheese
- 6 cups baby arugula
- 4 ½ cups cooked or canned chickpeas, rinsed and drained
- 1 ½ cups halved grape tomatoes
- 1 ¼ cups chopped kalamata olives
- ¾ cup chopped fresh parsley
- ½ cup balsamic vinegar

How to Prepare:

Combine the artichoke hearts, tomatoes, chickpeas, parsley, and olives in a bowl. Toss well to combine.

Drizzle the balsamic vinegar on top, then toss again to coat.

Add the arugula and toss again, then top with feta and serve right away.

Ginger, Tomato and Chickpea Bowl

Number of regular servings: 4

Calories per regular serving: 175

You will need:

- 300 grams canned chickpeas, rinsed and drained thoroughly
- 300 grams chopped tomatoes, juices reserved
- 1 large garlic clove, minced
- 1 spring onion, chopped
- ½ inch fresh ginger, peeled and minced
- 3 Tbsp low fat Greek yogurt
- 1 ½ Tbsp chopped fresh mint
- 1 ½ Tbsp chopped fresh coriander
- ¾ Tbsp olive oil
- 1 ½ tsp garam masala
- ¾ tsp mild curry paste
- Sea salt and freshly ground black pepper, to taste

How to Prepare:

Pour the dried chickpeas into a bowl, then pour in enough cold water to cover them by about an inch. Set aside to soak for 8 hours (overnight).

After soaking, drain the chickpeas, then transfer to a saucepan. Add enough cold water to cover them by about 2 inches. Boil over high flame for about 10 minutes, covered, then reduce to low flame and simmer for 1 hour, or until the chickpeas are tender. Add a pinch of salt, then drain and set aside.

Place a saucepan over medium flame and heat through. Once hot, add the oil and swirl to coat. And swirl to coat. Sauté the garlic and ginger with the garam masala, stirring for about 2 minutes.

Pour in the chickpeas and tomatoes, then simmer for 12 minutes.

In the meantime, combine the yogurt, mild curry paste, coriander, and mint in a serving bowl. Stir well, then season with salt and pepper to taste.

Add the chickpea and tomato mixture into the bowl, then stir gently to coat. Serve right away.

Roasted Tomato, Eggplant and Mozzarella

Number of regular servings: 6

Calories per regular serving: 240

You will need:

- 1 large eggplant
- 6 large tomatoes
- ¼ cup fresh basil leaves
- 4 Tbsp olive oil
- 4 Tbsp mozzarella cheese
- 2 tsp freshly squeezed lemon juice
- Sea salt and freshly ground black pepper, to taste

How to Prepare:

Set the grill over medium flame to preheat.

Slice the eggplant into long, thin pieces, then coat with olive oil. Grill for 3 minutes per side, or until tender and browned.

Slice the tomatoes thinly and grill for 2 minutes per side, or until tender. Lay the eggplant and tomato slices on a plate.

While hot, divide the mozzarella cheese on top of the roasted vegetables, then drizzle the lemon juice, basil, and olive oil all over.

Season to taste with salt and pepper, then serve right away.

Roasted Lemon Fennel with Olives

Number of regular servings: 6

Calories per regular serving: 230

You will need:

- 4 large fennel bulbs, trimmed, cored and quartered
- 2 cups green or black olives, pitted
- 1 ½ lemons
- ½ cup olive oil
- 3 Tbsp chopped fresh parsley
- Sea salt and freshly ground black pepper, to taste

How to Prepare:

Set the oven to 400 degrees F to preheat.

Lay the fennel quarters in a baking pan, cut side facing up. Add the olives and set aside.

Juice and zest the lemon, then pour both into a bowl. Add the olive oil, then season to taste with salt and pepper. Pour the mixture over the fennel and olives, then turn the fennel several times to coat.

Roast for 15 minutes, then stir again and roast for an additional 15 minutes, or until tender. Top with parsley, then serve right away.

Orange and Fennel Salad

Number of regular servings: 3

Calories per regular serving: 185

You will need:

- 2 small oranges, peeled and sliced into segments
- 1 small fennel bulb, trimmed and sliced thinly
- ½ red onion, sliced thinly
- 2 cups rocket leaves

For the dressing:

- 1 sun-dried tomato packed in oil, drained and chopped
- 1 small garlic clove, crushed
- 3 Tbsp extra virgin olive oil
- 1 ½ Tbsp pitted black olives, chopped
- 1/3 Tbsp chopped fresh parsley
- 1 ½ tsp balsamic vinegar

- Sea salt and freshly ground black pepper, to taste

How to Prepare:

Combine the olives, sun-dried tomato, parsley, garlic, and 1 tablespoon olive oil in a food processor. Blend until smooth, then transfer to a bowl.

Stir in the remaining olive oil, then add the vinegar and season to taste with salt and pepper. Set aside.

Place the orange slices into a bowl and add the rocket, fennel and onion. Toss well to combine, then add the dressing. Toss again until coated, then serve right away.

———————————————————————

Spiced Carrot and Parsnip Soup

Number of regular servings: 3

Calories per regular serving: 200

You will need:

- 2 parsnips, peeled, trimmed and chopped
- 2 carrots, peeled and chopped
- 1 small onion, minced
- 2 cups vegetable broth
- 1 ½ cups low fat milk
- 1 ½ Tbsp olive oil
- ¾ Tbsp curry powder
- 1 ½ tsp cumin seeds, toasted
- Sea salt and freshly ground black pepper, to taste

How to Prepare:

Place a saucepan over medium flame and heat through. Once hot, add the olive oil and swirl to coat.

Sauté the onion until translucent, then stir in the carrot and parsnip until combined. Cover and cook for 2 minutes, or until tender.

Add the curry powder and stir well to combine. Add the milk and vegetable broth, then season to taste with salt and pepper. Bring to a boil, then reduce to simmer. Simmer for 10 to 12 minutes, or until the carrot and parsnip are tender.

Turn off the heat and let cool, then blend in a food processor until smooth. Reheat over low flame, then ladle into bowls and top with toasted cumin seeds. Serve right away.

Moroccan Couscous and Veggie Bowl

Number of regular servings: 6

Calories per regular serving: 260

You will need:

- 2 medium onions, chopped
- 3 garlic cloves, crushed
- 300 grams canned chickpeas, rinsed and drained thoroughly
- 4 ½ cups vegetable broth
- 1 ½ cups cubed eggplant
- 1 ½ cups cubed zucchini
- 1 ½ cups easy cook couscous
- 1 cup peeled and cubed carrot
- 1/3 cup pureed tomatoes
- 1 ½ Tbsp olive oil
- 3 tsp ground cumin
- ¾ tsp ground ginger
- 1 ½ bay leaves

- Sea salt and freshly ground black pepper, to taste

How to Prepare:

Prepare the couscous based on package instructions. Set aside.

Place a large saucepan over medium flame and heat through. Add the oil and swirl to coat. Stir in the onion, carrot, spices, and garlic and sauté for about a minute.

Pour in the chickpeas, cubed eggplant and zucchini, then the pureed tomatoes and bay leaves. Add the stock and stir well to combine.

Cover and bring to a boil, then reduce to a simmer and cook for 8 minutes.

Fluff the couscous, then pour into a colander lined with cheese cloth to drain excess liquid.

Once drained, fold the couscous into the vegetables mixture and simmer until the sauce thickens. Adjust seasoning to taste.

Transfer the mixture into a bowl and fluff well. Serve right away.

Fattoush

Number of regular servings: 3

Calories per regular serving: 180

You will need:

- 3 tomatoes
- 3 spring onions
- 1 small green bell pepper, seeded and chopped
- ½ small cucumber, chopped
- 1 small garlic clove, crushed
- 2 Tbsp pitted and chopped Kalamata olives
- 2 Tbsp olive oil
- 1 ½ Tbsp freshly squeezed lemon juice
- 1 ½ Tbsp chopped fresh parsley
- 1 ½ Tbsp chopped fresh mint leaves
- 1 slice whole wheat bread, toasted
- Sea salt and freshly ground black pepper, to taste

How to Prepare:

Set the grill to medium flame to preheat.

Place the tomatoes into a baking dish and add enough boiling water to cover them by about half an inch. Set aside for 1 minute to become tender, then drain and skin.

Chop the tomatoes, then transfer to a food processor. Add the cucumber, spring onion, bell pepper, garlic, and lemon juice. Blend until pureed.

Pour the mixture into a bowl, then fold in the olive oil, mint, and parsley. Season to taste with salt and pepper.

Tear up the toasted slice of bread and place on top of the salad. Top with black olives, then serve right away.

Roasted Vegetable Salad

Number of regular servings: 6

Calories per regular serving: 240

You will need:

- 1 medium red onion, sliced into wedges
- 1 large eggplant, cubed
- 1 large zucchini, cubed
- 1 fennel bulb, trimmed and diced
- 2 red bell peppers, seeded and cubed
- 1 garlic bulb
- 4 Tbsp olive oil
- 4 Tbsp extra virgin olive oil
- 4 Tbsp pitted black olives
- 2 Tbsp chopped fresh basil
- 1 Tbsp chopped fresh sage
- 1 Tbsp chopped fresh thyme
- 2 tsp toasted pine nuts
- 2 tsp balsamic vinegar

- Sea salt and freshly ground black pepper

How to Prepare:

Set the oven to 450 degrees F to preheat.

Place the cubed eggplant and zucchini in a colander, then add a pinch of salt and toss well. Set aside for 30 minutes, then rinse and drain thoroughly. Blot dry with paper towels.

Place all the vegetables in a large mixing bowl, then add the sage, thyme, and olive oil. Toss to coat, then spread in a roasting pan. Spread out into an even layer.

Cut out a sheet of aluminum foil large enough to cover the garlic bulb. Place the bulb on top and add some oil, salt, and pepper. Seal tightly, then place in the roasting pan with the vegetables.

Roast for 45 minutes, or until the vegetables are browned and tender. Stir once every 15 minutes.

Transfer the bowl into a serving bowl.

Peel the aluminum foil carefully from the garlic, then discard the skin. Place in a bowl and add the extra virgin olive oil and balsamic vinegar. Crush the garlic, then mix well.

Pour the balsamic and garlic mixture over the vegetables, then add the basil, pine nuts, and olives. Toss well to combine, then serve right away.

Artichoke and Mushroom Soup

Number of regular servings: 6

Calories per regular serving: 250

You will need:

- 600 grams chestnut mushrooms, chopped
- 25 grams dried porcini mushrooms
- 1 large onion, chopped
- 2 garlic cloves, chopped
- 6 cups vegetable broth
- 4 cups Jerusalem artichokes
- 1 cup boiling water
- ½ cup dry sherry
- 3 Tbsp chopped toasted walnuts
- 1 ½ Tbsp chopped fresh thyme leaves
- 1 Tbsp grass-fed butter
- Sea salt and freshly ground black pepper, to taste

How to Prepare:

Place the dried porcini mushrooms into a bowl and add the boiling water. Soak for half an hour, then drain and save the soaking water.

Place a saucepan over medium flame and add the butter. Stir in the onion and thyme, then sauté for 10 minutes or until the onions are browned.

Increase to medium high flame, then add the chestnut and porcini mushrooms. Sauté for 2 minutes, then pour in the sherry and bring to a boil. Boil until the liquid is reduced.

Pour in the vegetable stock and mushroom soaking water. Bring to a boil, then cover and reduce to a simmer. Simmer for 20 minutes.

In the meantime, scrub and trim the artichokes, then peel and dice. Place a saucepan over medium flame and heat through. Add the oil and swirl to coat.

Sauté the artichokes and garlic for 10 minutes, or until the mixture is browned and tender.

Strain the mushroom soup in a pot, setting aside the solids in a bowl. Simmer the soup in a pot, then add the artichoke mixture.

Simmer for 20 minutes, or until the artichokes are tender. Turn off the heat and allow to cool slightly.

Blend the artichoke mixture in a food processor or using an immersion blender until pureed.

Pour the mixture back into the pot and stir in the mushroom mixture. Reheat over medium flame and season to taste with salt and pepper.

Ladle into soup bowls and top with toasted walnuts. Serve right away.

Roasted Garlicky Tomatoes

Number of regular servings: 9

Calories per regular serving: 185

You will need:

- 950 grams cherry tomatoes
- 9 slices whole wheat crusty bread, 1 day old
- 9 garlic cloves, diced
- 4 ½ Tbsp chopped fresh parsley
- Olive oil, as needed
- Sea salt and freshly ground black pepper, to taste

How to Prepare:

Set the oven to 425 degrees F to preheat.

Tear the bread and place in a food processor. Shred into crumbs, then transfer to a large skillet. Place over medium flame and toast all over until golden brown. Transfer to a plate.

Stir the diced garlic into the breadcrumb mixture, then fold in the parsley. Season with salt and pepper to taste, then mix well.

Spread the cherry tomatoes in a baking pan, then add the garlic breadcrumb mixture on top. Toss well to coat, then drizzle with olive oil.

Bake for 20 minutes, or until the crust is golden and the tomatoes are tender. Best served warm.

Split Pea and Carrot Curry

Number of regular servings: 3

Calories per regular serving: 260

You will need:

- 40 grams yellow split peas, soaked in cold water for 8 hours
- 2 large carrots, peeled and chopped
- 1 small potato, peeled and chopped
- 1 small onion, chopped
- 1 small garlic clove, chopped
- ½ red chili, seeded and chopped
- 4 cups cold water
- ¾ Tbsp sunflower oil
- ½ Tbsp butter, at room temperature
- 1 lime
- 1 tsp chopped fresh coriander
- 1 tsp hot curry paste
- ¾ tsp grated fresh ginger

- Sea salt and freshly ground black pepper, to taste

How to Prepare:

Drain the split peas thoroughly, then rinse under cold running water and drain. Transfer to a saucepan, then add 4 cups cold water and bring to a boil over high flame.

Boil for 10 minutes, then reduce to low flame and simmer for 30 minutes or until the split peas are tender.

In the meantime, combine the butter and coriander. Juice and zest the lime, then stir both into the butter mixture. Season to taste with black pepper and mix well.

Line a small bowl with aluminum foil, then pour the butter mixture into the bowl. Refrigerate to chill until solid.

Place a saucepan over medium flame and add the oil. Swirl to coat, then sauté the onion, garlic, ginger, and chili for 10 minutes or until browned. Add the curry paste, potato, and carrot, then sauté for 5 minutes.

Pour the curry mixture into the saucepan of split peas. Stir well, then bring to a boil. Once boiling, reduce to a simmer and cover. Simmer for 25 minutes, or until the vegetables are tender.

Turn off the heat and allow to cool slightly. Once cooled, blend until smooth using an immersion blender or food processor. Season to taste with salt and pepper, then reheat over medium flame.

Before serving, ladle the soup into bowls. Take out the herb butter and slice. Place a pat of the herb butter into each bowl and serve right away.

Chapter 7 – Snack Recipes

Zesty Baked Apples

Number of regular servings: 4

Calories per regular serving: 163

You will need:

- 4 baking apples
- 4 dried dates, minced
- 4 dried apricots, diced
- ½ cup chopped almonds
- 5 Tbsp nonfat Greek yogurt
- 2 tsp raw honey
- 2 tsp mixed spice
- 2 oranges

How to Prepare:

Set the oven to 400 degrees F to preheat.

Combine the chopped dates and apricots in a bowl with the honey, almonds, and mixed spice. Juice the oranges, then stir into the mixture. Set aside.

Core the apples without removing the bottom section. Spoon the zesty mixture into the apples, then place on a baking dish. Pour some boiling water around the apples into the dish, the cover tightly with foil.

Bake for 45 minutes, or until the apples are tender. Transfer to a cooling rack and carefully remove the foil.

Transfer the baked apples on a serving dish and add a dollop of yogurt on top. Serve right away.

Warm Avocado, Grapefruit and Endive Snacks

Number of regular servings: 6

Calories per regular serving: 225

You will need:

- 3 avocados, halved and pitted
- 1 ½ pink grapefruits, peeled and sliced into small segments
- 1 ½ fresh limes
- 3 cups chopped endives
- ¾ cup chopped shallots
- 3 Tbsp olive oil
- 3 Tbsp chopped fresh parsley
- Sea salt and freshly ground black pepper, to taste

How to Prepare:

Set the oven to 425 degrees F to preheat.

Place a skillet over medium high flame and heat through. Once hot, add the oil and swirl to coat. And swirl to coat.

Sauté the shallots and endives until tender and browned. Stir in the parsley, then season with salt and pepper to taste.

Arrange the halved avocados, cut side facing up, on a baking sheet. Spoon the endive mixture into the cavity of each, then bake for 12 minutes or until the avocado is slightly browned and tender.

Transfer to a platter and add the grapefruit. Squeeze lime juice over the avocados, then serve right away.

Banana and Dark Chocolate Sandwiches

Number of regular servings: 6

Calories per regular serving: 318

You will need:

- 12 slices sourdough or sprouted wheat bread
- 3 large bananas, sliced into thin rounds
- 6 oz dark chocolate, diced
- ½ Tbsp raw honey

How to Prepare:

Place six bread slices on a platter and divide the banana slices on top of each.

Spoon the dark chocolate over the banana slices, then drizzle the honey on top.

Place another slice of bread over each, then toast for 4 minutes, or until the bread is crisp and the chocolate is melted.

Transfer to a plate and let stand for 3 minutes to cool slightly. Best served warm.

Peanut Butter Muffins

Number of regular servings: 18

Calories per regular serving: 184

You will need:

- 2 eggs
- 1 ¼ cups whole wheat pastry flour
- 1 ¼ creamy peanut butter
- ¾ cup rolled oats
- ¾ cup plain Greek yogurt
- 1/3 cup wheat germ
- ¾ cup unsweetened applesauce
- 4 ½ Tbsp raw honey
- 4 ½ Tbsp dark brown sugar
- 3 tsp pure vanilla extract
- 1 ½ tsp baking powder
- ¾ tsp baking soda
- ¾ tsp ground cinnamon
- 1/3 tsp fine sea salt

How to Prepare:

Set the oven to 375 degrees F to preheat. Line 18 muffin tins with paper liners and set aside.

In a large bowl, combine the oats, flour, wheat germ, cinnamon, baking soda, baking powder, and salt. Set aside.

In a separate bowl, combine the applesauce, peanut butter, sugar, honey, vanilla, and eggs. Add the Greek yogurt and mix well.

Fold the flour mixture into the peanut butter mixture, then mix well until combined.

Divide the batter among the prepared muffin tins, then bake for 18 minutes or until firm and golden brown.

Set on a cooling rack and let cool completely. Serve right away or store in an airtight container and serve after 24 hours for better flavor.

Cayenne Trail Mix

Number of regular servings: 15 (30 grams each)

Calories per regular serving: 154

You will need:

- ½ cup almonds
- ½ cup Brazil nuts
- ½ cup cashews
- ½ cup pistachio nuts
- ½ cup raisins
- ½ cup dried berries, such as cranberries or raspberries
- 1 ½ tsp olive oil
- 1 ½ tsp chopped fresh rosemary
- 1 ½ tsp cayenne powder
- ½ tsp garlic powder

How to Prepare:

Set the oven to 400 degrees F to preheat. Spread all the nuts on a rimmed baking sheet, then drizzle the oil on top.

Sprinkle the rosemary, garlic powder, and cayenne pepper on top, then toss well to coat. Roast for 10 minutes.

After 10 minutes, stir in the dried berries and raisins. Stir and roast for an additional 5 minutes.

Transfer to a cooling rack, then allow to cool. Transfer to an airtight container and store in a cool, dry shelf for up to 7 days.

Spiced Roasted Chickpeas

Number of regular servings: 6

Calories per regular serving: 150

You will need:

- 24 oz canned chickpeas, rinsed and drained thoroughly
- 1 ½ tsp olive oil
- ¾ tsp garlic powder
- ¾ tsp onion
- ¾ tsp organic buffalo wing sauce
- 1/3 tsp smoked paprika
- 1/3 tsp onion powder
- 1/3 tsp cumin
- 1/3 tsp sea salt
- ¼ tsp cayenne pepper

How to Prepare:

Set the oven to 425 degrees F to preheat. Line a baking sheet with parchment paper and set aside.

Combine all the spices in a bowl and set aside.

Blot the chickpeas dry with paper towels, then spread them on the prepared baking sheet. Sprinkle the spice mixture over the chickpeas and toss well to coat.

Bake for 25 minutes, or until the chickpeas are crisp. Stir once every 10 minutes.

Transfer to a cooling rack and let cool slightly before serving.

Fruity Oat Bars

Number of regular servings: 24 (1 piece each)

Calories per regular serving: 113

You will need:

- 3 eggs
- 1 ½ cups whole wheat flour
- ½ cup steel cut oats
- ½ cup low fat milk
- 1/3 cup raisins
- 1/3 cup raw honey
- ¼ cup chopped almonds
- 2 ½ Tbsp melted grass-fed butter
- 1 ½ tsp mixed spice
- 2 oranges

How to Prepare:

Set the oven is 400 degrees F to preheat. Line a large baking sheet with parchment paper and set aside.

Whisk the eggs with the milk and honey in a bowl. Sift in the whole wheat flour, then add the oats, raisins, almonds, butter, and mixed spice.

Juice the oranges, then stir the mixture into the batter. Pour into the prepared baking sheet.

Bake for 20 to 25 minutes, or until firm. Transfer to a wire rack and allow to cool completely.

Slice into 24 equal rectangles, then serve right away. Alternatively, refrigerate and serve chilled.

_____

Almond Raspberry Yogurt Bowls

Number of regular servings: 6

Calories per regular serving: 207

You will need:

- 15 oz frozen raspberries

- 3 cups Greek yogurt

- 1/3 cup brown sugar

- 4 ½ Tbsp raw honey

- 3 Tbsp freshly grated orange zest

- 3 Tbsp sliced almonds

- ¾ tsp almond extract

How to Prepare:

Combine the sugar and raspberries in a saucepan, then place over medium flame and bring to a simmer.

Cook for 10 minutes, then stir and set aside until cooled slightly. Transfer to the refrigerator and let chill for 15 minutes.

Meanwhile, combine the honey, yogurt, orange zest, and almond extract in a bowl. Stir until combined.

Take the raspberry mixture out of the refrigerator and fold 2 cups into the yogurt mixture until just combined with a swirling effect.

Divide the mixture among six bowls, then spoon the remaining raspberry mixture on top. Add the almonds, then serve right away.

Nutty Cherry Bombs

Number of regular servings: 6

Calories per regular serving: 276

You will need:

- ¾ cup slivered almonds
- ¾ cup chopped walnuts
- 1/3 cup dried dark cherries, unsweetened
- 1/3 cups dried pitted dates
- 1 ½ Tbsp almond butter
- 1/3 tsp ground cinnamon
- Sea salt, to taste

How to Prepare:

Pour the almond and walnuts into a food processor, then pulse until finely ground.

Add the almond butter, cinnamon, dates, cherries, and a pinch of salt, then blend until pasty.

Divide the mixture into two tablespoon servings, then roll into balls. Place on a tray and serve right away. Alternatively, refrigerate for at least half an hour and serve chilled.

Soft Almond Cookies

Number of regular servings: 30 (1 cookie each)

Calories per regular serving: 130

You will need:

- 2 small eggs
- 1 ½ cups all-purpose flour
- 1 ½ cups almond meal
- ¾ cup unsalted grass-fed butter
- ½ cup muscovado sugar
- 1 ½ tsp almond extract
- ¾ tsp baking soda
- 1/6 tsp fine sca salt

How to Prepare:

Set the oven to 375 degrees F to preheat. Line two large baking sheets with parchment paper and set aside.

Sift the all-purpose and almond flours with the bicarbonate of soda into a bowl, then sift in the salt. Cut in the butter and rub until the mixture becomes crumbly.

Add the sugar and eggs, then mix well until thoroughly combined.

Lightly flour a clean work surface, then place the dough on top. Roll out into a sheet, then cut into cookie rounds.

Arrange the cookies on the prepared baking sheets spaced at least an inch apart.

Bake the cookies for 12 minutes, or until golden brown. Place on a cooling rack and let stand for 5 minutes, then serve.

Cilantro and Hummus Quesadillas

Number of regular servings: 6

Calories per regular serving: 193

You will need:

- 3 large whole wheat pitas, halved crosswise
- 3 jarred roasted red bell peppers, drained and chopped
- 1 ½ cups baby spinach leaves

For the cilantro hummus:

- 2 small garlic cloves, peeled
- 1 ¼ cups cooked chickpeas or rinsed and drained canned chickpeas
- 1/3 cup fresh cilantro
- 3 Tbsp water
- 1 ½ Tbsp extra virgin olive oil
- 1 ½ Tbsp freshly squeezed lime juice

How to Prepare:

Set the oven to 350 degrees F to preheat.

Meanwhile, combine the garlic and cilantro in a food processor and blend until shredded.

Pour in the chickpeas, olive oil, lime juice, and water, then blend until creamy and smooth. Set aside.

Lay the halved pita on a baking sheet, then spread the hummus over the pita.

Lay the spinach and bell peppers on top, then bake for 1 minutes, or until the pita is crisp.

Transfer to a platter, slice into wedges, then serve right away.

Zesty Poached Pears

Number of regular servings: 3

Calories per regular serving: 90

You will need:

- 3 pears, peeled
- 1 ½ tsp raw honey
- 2 ½ Tbsp freshly squeezed orange juice
- 2 ½ Tbsp freshly squeezed lemon juice
- ½ cinnamon stick
- ½ star anise

How to Prepare:

Arrange the pears in a pan, then pour the orange and lemon juices on top. Add the honey, star anise, and cinnamon stick.

Add about ½ cup of water, then cover and place over high flame. Bring to a boil, then reduce to a simmer. Simmer for 15 minutes. Uncover and simmer for 5 minutes, or until the pears are tender and the sauce is thickened.

Serve right away. Alternatively, refrigerate for at least 30 minutes, then serve chilled.

_____

Conclusion

Thank you again for downloading this book!

I hope this book was able to help you achieve your health and fitness goals with the 5:2 Diet.

The next step is to apply all of the knowledge that you have gained from this book. Launching your personalized meal plan can start any time. All you have to do is print it out and post it on your refrigerator wall. Then, gather your tools and ingredients, whip up your meals, and you are all set! Don't forget to include exercise into your regimen so that you will not only lose weight, but also develop an overall strong and resilient physique.

Finally, if you enjoyed this book, then I'd like to ask you for a favor, would you be kind enough to leave a review for this book on Amazon? It'd be greatly appreciated!

Thank you and good luck!